Essential Oils for Pets

Simple but amazingly effective natural remedies that will improve the health and well-being of your pet!

By: Julie Summers

© **Copyright 2015 by Julie Summers - All rights reserved.**

This document is geared towards providing exact and reliable information in regards to the topic and issue covered. The publication is sold with the idea that the publisher is not required to render accounting, officially permitted, or otherwise, qualified services. If advice is necessary, legal or professional, a practiced individual in the profession should be ordered.

- From a Declaration of Principles which was accepted and approved equally by a Committee of the American Bar Association and a Committee of Publishers and Associations.

In no way is it legal to reproduce, duplicate, or transmit any part of this document in either electronic means or in printed format. Recording of this publication is strictly prohibited and any storage of this document is not allowed unless with written permission from the publisher. All rights reserved.

The information provided herein is stated to be truthful and consistent, in that any liability, in terms of inattention or otherwise, by any usage or abuse of any policies, processes, or directions contained within is the solitary and utter responsibility of the recipient reader. Under no circumstances will any legal responsibility or blame be held against the publisher for any reparation, damages, or monetary loss due to the information herein, either directly or indirectly.

Respective authors own all copyrights not held by the publisher.

The information herein is offered for informational purposes solely, and is universal as so. The presentation of the information is without contract or any type of guarantee assurance.

The trademarks that are used are without any consent, and the publication of the trademark is without permission or backing by the trademark owner. All trademarks and brands within this book are for clarifying purposes only and are the owned by the owners themselves, not affiliated with this document.

Essential Oils for Pets

Introduction

Chapter 1 – What is Essential Oil?

- Essential oils are natural remedies
- Essential oils benefit you
- Save yourself some money
- Essential oils are safe
- Essential oils are easy to use and apply

Chapter 2 – Fundamental principles of using essential oils

- Dilution of Essential Oils
- Application Methods of Essential Oils
- Using Essential Oils Aromatically
- Using Essential Oils Topically
- Using Essential Oils Internally

Chapter 3 – Acceptable essential oil for your pets

- Roman Chamomile Oil.
- Rosemary Oil.
- Peppermint & Fennel.

- Lavender.
- Tea Tree Oil.
- Dilution Ratios for Pets.

Chapter 4 – Tips for successful application

- Zoopharmacognosy of Essential Oils
- Use Essential Oils with Respect
- Understand Your Pet's Responses
- Testing Your Pet's Responses
- Other tips for safe use of essential oils include:

Chapter 5 – Shopping guide for Essential oil

Conclusion

Introduction

I want to thank you and congratulate you for purchasing the book, "Essential oils for pets".

You are probably like myself, seeing your pet as one of your family members. You want to offer them the best that you can in terms of caring for them. Doing what you can to make sure that their overall well-being is good and healthy is important to you and that is why you are reading this book today.

You will be glad that you decided to purchase this book because you are going to be learning a lot of different ways that you can naturally look after you four-legged friend in a safe and non-toxic way. Unfortunately in today's world there are so many products out there that are filled with harmful toxins that cannot only harm us, but harm our pets as well. It is important that we as responsible pet owners do our part to ensure that we are providing our pets with healthy remedies to their everyday common ailments such as ticks and fleas. You will be given treatments in this book using essential oils to battle against these problems that arise with your loving pets.

Many of us have hectic busy lives in this fast-paced world we live in, so the idea of making our own tick and flea treatments, and pet shampoo can seem a bit challenging. This may seem like too much effort to do when there are pet products on the market which are ready made. The problem with many products on the market today is that many artificial products have a wide range of chemicals in them that are not only harmful to our dear pets but also the environment.

It is important that you decide whether you want to take the chance that some artificial product you use on your pet ends up being banned down the road due to the high levels of harmful toxins in it. Are you sure you are willing to put your pet's health and well-being at risk?

The sad reality of the situation in our world is that there are manufacturers that do cut corners. They may not use chemicals and additives that are known to be harmful, but they could be using chemical compounds that are not fully understood or have not been properly tested for long-term effects. These compounds could take years before they start showing their darker side in side effects, then it could be too late.

Learning to make your own natural pet products will be a much healthier alternative for your pet than the commercial products, many of which contain toxic substances. It is not worth the risk of your pet's health. Going for the natural remedies is the better and safer choice. We want our pets to be with us as long as possible living healthy happy lives so this is why we are looking into using natural remedies. It may be surprising to you, but many of the essential oil treatments for our pets have similar benefits for humans.

These home remedies are going to be a lot easier not only on your pet but also on the environment as well. Essential oils are so concentrated you will find that a little will certainly go a long way. I know that you want to do what is right in the type of treatments you are using on your pet. You are going to find the natural treatments offered in this book wonderful, yet simple to put together and apply. I wish you and your pet great success with the use of these natural essential oils pet treatments!

Chapter 1 – What is Essential Oil?

Why use essential oils? What are essential oils? Are they really useful and important?

Essential oils are concentrated liquids that are extracted from a plant during distillation. These can be described as the essence of the plant itself and contain the chemically active components of the plant. It is basically just a very concentrated plant essence.

The name essential oil is something of a misnomer because these essences are not actual oils, though they do exhibit some of the properties of oils - for example, they will float on water.

It is important to know the botanical name of the plant, its origin, the extraction method used and also what the basic chemical components of the essential oil is. Oils extracted in different parts of the world, even from the same species, may have a different chemical makeup. It is also important to find out what distillation method was used as this can also have an effect.

Most essential oils are extracted from particular parts of the plants such as the leaves, seed, twigs, flowers, roots, berries, citrus peels, woods barks, depending where the essence to be collected is strongest. It takes great numbers of plants just to manufacture essential oils because the oils are so concentrated. Because they are so concentrated, they are amazingly powerful healers - with essential oils you measure the dosage in drops, not teaspoons. One small bottle can heal a number of different ailments, not only in humans, but also in pets.

The ancient Egyptians were believed to be the first people to use essential oils. They understood the power of the oils and used them as part of their healing rituals. The essential oils were treated as very precious items - so exquisite that only royals and priests were allowed to use them. Other nationalities such as the Greeks, Chinese, and Romans also used essential oils and some of herbs for aromatherapy, personal hygiene uses, and treatment of various ailments and illnesses. Essential oils are still popular to this day because of their amazing properties in healing.

Now, going back to our question, "Why use essential oils?" There are lots of reasons why, but here are some of the more important ones.

Essential oils are natural remedies

They are naturally grown, collected, and obtained from plants. These are plants that usually contain some of the most powerful healing components, which are quite useful and powerful in terms of treating ailments.

Essential oils benefit you

They offer a natural alternative to dangerous artificial chemical or commercially- produced remedies, many of which have nasty side effects. Quality essential oils are helpful in treating ailments such as memory loss, congestion, pain, headaches, inflammation, and nausea. They are also helpful in stimulating the immune system, aiding in killing viruses, bacteria and fungus, as well as various other skin ailments. The benefits are not just seen in humans though, but also in pets. By using the right combination of oils you create a powerful healing and restorative remedy.

Save yourself some money

Another reason why you should use essential oils is because commercially available medicines are quite expensive. You can actually make your own essential oils at home saving you more money because plants containing essential oils can be home grown and planted everywhere.

Essential oils are safe

Essential oils, when used correctly, will not harm you or your pet. Moreover, the oils have very few side effects at all. Unfortunately, the same cannot be said of commercially available medications - many of which cause side effects that are just as bad as the symptoms of the illness being treated. The key is in doing your research into the properties of the oils and choosing the best one to treat your pet's particular ailment.

Essential oils are easy to use and apply

The application of essential oils on your pets is very similar to how you apply them to yourself. Your pets can inhale the oils just as you do or the oils may be applied, diluted, directly to the affected area. They are also highly valuable and helpful when it comes to training your pets as they help them concentrate and focus. The oils can also help to treat anxiety issues in pets.

Chapter 2 – Fundamental principles of using essential oils

Essential oils are remarkably effective in treating various conditions in pets and in maintaining the overall wellbeing of the pets. The oils are not only cost-effective but also easy to use and can be used even by people with little knowledge of the oils as long as the person is passionate about learning the basic guidelines. At the basic level, anyone can follow three core guidelines to use essential oils effectively and safely in pets.

The three guidelines are:

1. **Personal judgment:** Your judgment of the situation is one of the most important yardsticks of mastering the successful use of essential oils in your pets. You have to learn to observe your pet, take note of various psychological, physical and cosmetic problems, and trust your instinct and the prescriptions of your vet. If you can build your personal judgment, then you can learn how to use essential oils in your pets quickly and fruitfully.

2. **Safe is not necessarily foolproof**: While the essential oils used in pets are typically safe and potent, you should never consider them absolutely fail-safe. Just as pure drinking water can harm the body when used in excess, the oils can harm your pets if you do not use them appropriately. Therefore, you should assess your pets thoroughly, identify their sensitivities and allergies, and apply the right precautionary measures when diluting or administering essential oils to the pets. In fact, it is advisable to start with small dosages and conservative applications of the oils and to monitor how your pets respond before you can increase the dosages.

3. **Follow precautions strictly**: All the recommendations and techniques for using essential oils in pets usually come with related precautions. Following these precautions will not only help you to safeguard the overall health of your pet but also to achieve your cherished goals quickly. It is important to know that the oils will take time to yield desired results and to use common sense when applying the oils. And as a rule, it is vital to start conservatively, using less oil first and never overdoing any application.

Dilution of Essential Oils

Proper dilution of essential oils is critical to avoid causing adverse reactions in the pets. For instance, if citrus oils are not diluted properly, the pet's skin becomes increasingly sensitive to natural light or ultraviolet radiation. Most essential oils are diluted with a carrier or base oil before being applied to a pet. The best carrier or base oil is organic fractionated coconut oil, grape-seed oil or cold-pressed olive oil. But if your pet is allergic to nuts, make sure to avoid using nut oil as a carrier.

When diluting essential oil make sure to consider the weight of your pet. Treat a small pet weighing less than 20 pounds as you would treat a human baby or toddler and dilute the oil for application on the pet by 30-90% depending on the pet's size.

For application of oils on larger pets, dilute as you would for adult human usage. But just as is done with humans it is important to start with highly diluted oils before reducing the dilution as treatment progresses. Moreover, most essential oils usually detoxify the pet's body at the cellular level and cause the expulsion of toxins via body organs and so giving highly diluted oil will prevent overloading the pet with detoxification.

As a rule, dilute 1 drop of essential oil with 10 drops of base/carrier oil. And if the oil gets into the eye of your pet, rinse gently with the base/carrier oil. Never use water. Besides, branded essential oils usually come with recognizable symbols for indicating how much dilution you should perform. The symbols are:

GREEN: The oil is safe and can be used as directed without dilution.

ORANGE: The oil requires moderate dilution for safe use.

RED: The oil requires heavier dilution/precautions for safe use.

Application Methods of Essential Oils

Every essential oil must be applied properly in order to elicit the desired response in the pet. Typically, you can apply a few drops of essential oil on location, add a drop or two on the pets paws, or have the pet smelling the oil right out of a bottle. You may also choose to diffuse the oil next to your sleeping pet, massage the pet's legs with the oil when it seems to be experiencing pain, or drop calming oil on your pet's paws whenever you expect visitors. The possibilities are countless.

Some oils such as peppermint and lemon have more than one application method while some such as wintergreen oil has only one application method. Since applying the oil wrongly may cause adverse reactions in your pet, it is prudent to research the oil you intend to use and learn how to apply it properly. As you research, you should take note of usage recommendations, dilution and application methods. If an essential oil is not for internal application, never try to use it that way.

There are four major application methods for essential oils in pets.

- Topically
- Internally
- Aromatically
- Externally (such as around the room/home)

Using Essential Oils Aromatically

Because of their amazingly good smell, essential oils have been used as deodorizers and fresheners for many decades.

And it is due to the good smell that aromatic application has been widely popular. But there is more of the good smell than what ordinarily meets the eye! When inhaled, the active ingredients in the essential oils are usually processed by the pet's olfactory bulb or limbic system within the brain, resulting in desirable responses.

Aromatic application is:

- Nurturing to the pets respiratory system, including sinuses.

- Protects the pet against airborne contaminants.

- Capable of relaying active ingredients into the pet's bloodstream, promoting the health and well-being of the pet in multiple ways.

- Supportive to the pet's hormonal system, moods and tension.

- The aroma that is breathed in by the pet during an aromatic application is a fine vapor or mist of the oil which has the same medicinal properties as the oil itself. And since the olfactory system of the pet is closely linked to its limbic system, application of the oil aromatically results in positive psychological and physical effects.

There are different types of aromatic applications, such as:

Direct Inhalation: When you want to calm or ground your pet, direct inhalation of an effective essential oil comes in handy. You can simply add a drop or two of the oil into your hand and then cupping the hand before the nose or mouth of the pet. Alternatively, you can hold a bottle of the essential oil an inch or so from the pet's nose to allow the pet to breathe in the aroma. Opening and closing the bottle of oil will expose the oil to air and increase its oxidative state, allowing you to use less oil throughout the day. Nevertheless, some essential oils such as Cinnamon or Oregano should be properly diluted prior to direct inhalation.

Indirect Inhalation: When you intend to ensure deeper and better sleep for your pet, you can apply Vetiver indirectly. Add a drop or two of the oil to a cotton ball, handkerchief, shirt collar, pillow case, hair or small fabric and bring the item close to the pet's nose and mouth so that the pet can breathe in the oil's aroma.

Diffusing the Oil: With a good diffuser that operates at room temperature/cool air or at ultrasonic vibrations to send molecules of the oil into the air, you can keep oil molecules in air for long and allow the pet to breathe in the aroma.

Humidification: Cool humidifiers will keep oil molecules air-bound for many hours. However, you should choose the best plastic components for humidification because oil molecules can damage plastics such as PEEK, ULTEM, and KYNAR.

Fan/Vent: Similar to indirect inhalation, the oil can be added to a piece of cloth and placed in front of a fan or vent so that the aroma from the cloth can reach the pet. Ginger and peppermint for calming motion sickness in pets can be applied in this manner.

Cologne/ Perfume Smells: Add 1-2 drops of the oil behind the pet's ears, or add 1-3 drops of the oil to alcohol and use the mixture to mist the pets body/fur.

While applying essential oils aromatically is easy and safe, you should monitor closely how the pet responds to the oil to avoid overwhelming the pet's system or causing sensitivity/ allergic reactions.

Using Essential Oils Topically

Topical application is more delicate but fairly easy. While most essential oils can be applied topically, usage varies from oil to oil and according to the frequency and degree of dilution. Prior to topical application, it is prudent to assess and know your do$ skin type. If the skin is highly sensitive, then you should always dilute oil before applying on the skin. If you are not sure about your pet's skin type, you should perform a patch test. As a precaution, prioritize dilution. It will not diminish the effectiveness of the oil and will most likely boost its absorption by preventing evaporation. Dilution will also reduce negative skin reactions.

Most essential oil brands for topical use come with simple visual guides on how to use them. The guides include:

NEAT: Means the oil can be applied directly to the pet's skin without dilution.

SENSITIVE: Means that the oil can be applied directly without dilution, but must be diluted before use if the pet has a sensitive skin. Dilute in the ratio of (1 drop of oil: 3 drops of carrier).

DILUTE: Means the oil is very potent and may cause irritation on any skin type, so it must be properly diluted before use.

The most popular topical applications include:

Massage: Massage the joints, tissues and muscles of the pet with the oil.

Apply over the area concerned: Apply the oil directly over the abdomen, chest, back of the neck or any other area that has the condition to be treated.

Apply over reflex points: Add the oil directly to the pet's reflex points of the arms, toes and ears, especially if the pet has a sensitive skin and you want to avoid irritation.

Foot baths/bathing: You can add your essential oil in a bathwater, mix it carefully with the carrier and then soak the foot/body of the pet in the mixture. Malaleuca foot baths usually help to soothe itchy feet.

Precautions to consider during topical applications include:

If you apply citrus oil and other phototoxic oils topically, avoid exposing the pet to sunlight within 12 hours of the application. In fact, such oils should be applied in the evening or to the area of the pet's body that will not experience direct sun-exposure.

Every pet is different and so even the gentlest oil can cause adverse reaction in some pets. Therefore, know your pet's skin type and prioritize dilution.

Never apply excess oil on the pet's skin even if a previous application showed no adverse reaction.

It is wiser to layer the oils than to blend them. So, apply one oil first, wait for some minutes/hours before you apply another instead of blending many oils and applying at once.

Using Essential Oils Internally

Internal usage of the oils requires greater care. Usually, some oils are benign and will not cause adverse reactions, but some are less benign and may cause some problems in your pets. When you plan to use the oils internally for your pets, remember.

Less is more: Start off small, see how it works with your pet before you increase the quantity.

More Frequency before more drops: Your pet's liver will tolerate small doses of the oils well. Therefore, it is wiser to give a single drop after 30-90 minutes instead of 3-4 drops at once.

Save internal application till when you need it most: Often, a massage on the pet's belly with digestive oil will improve the condition and should be first choice instead of internal application.

Limit the number of daily drops: Generally, your pet should not consume more than 25 drops of any oil per day.

Some oils require more caution than others when you use them internally: For instance, essential oils that have high quantities of phenols (such as cinnamon, oregano and thyme) must be used with more care because they generally accumulate in the pets' liver and may cause liver function problems.

Prioritize dilution for oils you intend to apply internally: Make sure to dilute essential oils for internal application with edible carriers such as olive oil or coconut oil to reduce potential irritation of the pet's mucous membranes.

If your pet is pregnant, nursing, has liver issues or compromised immunity, or has a major health problem, you should avoid internal application unless advised to do so by a competent vet or pet naturopathic expert.

Every essential oil brand typically comes with instructions as to whether it can be used internally. Therefore, make sure to read the User Manual carefully when you purchase essential oils for your pets.

The most popular internal applications of essential oil include:

Cooking: Several essential oils (such as oregano and rosemary) for pets can be baked or cooked before oral administration. Prepared as part of certain recipes, a few drops of the oil is added to other ingredients to form a potent meal for the pet. Make sure to start with small drops of the oil and to increase the drops depending on observed response.

Nevertheless, all essential oils must be applied internally with moderation, regardless of whether they are cooked or baked.

Drinking: Many essential oils (including lemon, peppermint and cinnamon) can be added to the pet's drinking water or milk. For instance, for single uses, a drop of essential oil should be added to a minimum of 4 Oz of almond milk, rice milk or water before drinking. While water and oil will never mix, you can blend them carefully by stirring so that the pet finds the blend drinkable. However, you must avoid adding essential oil to non-oil based liquids that can irritate mucous membranes.

Supplementation: Pets can also be given essential oils as supplements in their meals. For instance, you can purchase branded essential oil supplements for immunity, energy, digestion and fatty acids, and then add to their meals as necessary.

Rectal/Vaginal Insertions: Vaginal and rectal insertions of essential oils should only be attempted under the advice and supervision of a pet naturopath. The oils used must be diluted first and must be applied with extreme caution.

Chapter 3 – Acceptable essential oil for your pets

Using the essential oil treatments in this book regularly will help to keep your pets in the best shape in terms of health. Below are some oils that are used in general functions, by giving them a try you will soon get to know the ones that your pet enjoys and which ones they may not be too fond of. The oils listed here are used for the general good health of your pets. But just remember that one of the best ways to help to keep your pet healthy is making sure to have regular interaction with them. It is important to remember to use therapeutic grade oils on your pets not perfume quality or aromatherapy grade oils.

These can do more harm than good for your pet because they are distilled using solvents or are adulterated. Pure therapeutic essential oils are steam distilled and do not contain chemicals.

Make a point of putting some time aside to use perhaps in taking your pet for a walk this will please them, and get you both out for some exercise as well as time to strengthen your bonds with your pet. Your pets want so much to please you they love you unconditionally so show them that they are special by making sure to offer them large doses of attention and affection these will help keep their health and spirits up.

Providing your pet with attention is very vital in their well-being; they will be less stressed and happier if you are showing them love and attention. Keep them in top shape and use aromatherapy treatments to help keep them feeling happy and healthy.

Roman Chamomile Oil.

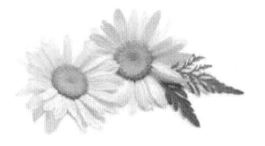

Roman Chamomile oil is a natural analgesic and sedative. You must never apply it neat. You can mix it with two tablespoons of olive oil and a few drops of lavender oil and a few drops of Roman Chamomile. Give your pet a tummy rub with it just before bedtime—this will help you to both sleep better. If your pet is suffering from flatulence or they have eaten a big meal apply it after the pet has eaten it will help get rid of the flatulence.

Rosemary Oil.

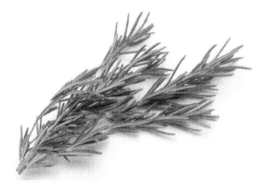

Rosemary oil can be used on both pets and cats. Rosemary oil is great to help boost your pet's immune system, and also to give them some pep, help to lift their spirits up. It is a great oil for helping fight against anti-fungal, and anti-bacterial, it is a great anti-viral oil. It is also good in helping to relieve stiff joints and muscles.

Peppermint & Fennel.

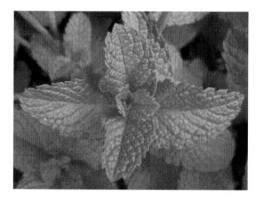

These work well on pets, but do not use them on cats. These oils can help to ease digestion and are perfect for that special tummy rub. The peppermint oil has analgesic properties and helps to battle against parasites. Giving your pet a daily tummy rub with two tablespoons of olive oil and a few drops of peppermint and fennel oil mixed well together will make a good tummy rub. The tummy rub will help keep your pet worms free.

Lavender.

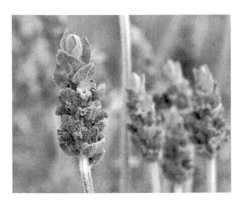

Lavender oil is used in remedies throughout this book. It is known to some as the most useful essential oil. It is an oil that you can use on pets and cats it will help you to prevent a wide range of ailments that your pet may suffer from.

It is an oil that is anti-viral, anti-fungal, and anti-bacterial and is also great in helping to balance just about every internal system within your pets body. It is a mild analgesic, and has anti-inflammatory properties as well. You can also use it to treat minor burns, scrapes, and cuts. Lavender can help to disinfect a minor cut or scrape that your pet may have.

If your poor pet is suffering from sunburn use some lavender to help to soothe it.

At night time to help your cat relax place a drop of lavender at the base of your cat's neck while you are cuddling with him/her, this will help them to relax and sleep better.

Blend a few drops of lavender oil with two tablespoons or so of olive oil depending on size of pet you may want to add less or more olive oil. Then, apply this nightly to your pet's tummy it will help make them calmer and happier.

The great thing about lavender oil is it is nice and gentle and you can blend it with any other oils. If you have a neurotic cat or pet, this is a good choice in oils to keep handy. It will have a wonderful calming effect on your pet's mind. It is also very good at calming humans, try putting a few drops on your inner pillowcase to help you sleep better. So you, and your pet can both have a calm night's sleep.

Tea Tree Oil.

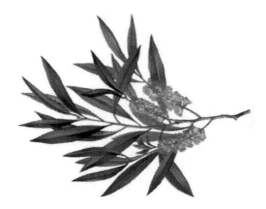

Never use tea tree oil on your cat as this could kill your cat, you should also avoid using it on small pets. If your pet is less than ten pounds I would not use tea tree oil on it. Some vets believe it is toxic to use while others say if it is diluted properly it is not toxic. If you do not feel comfortable using it I would leave it out of your pet remedies.

Dilution Ratios for Pets.

The best way to figure out the dilution ratio is to use your pet's weight as a guide. A pet that is one hundred pounds will be able to tolerate a lot more than a pet that weighs less than 25 pounds. Basically you will be adding less essential oils with and more carrier oil such as olive oil, coconut oil, or almond oil, the less the pet weighs. If your pet weighs less than ten pounds, then you would be looking at a ratio of 1:100 or one drop of essential oils to the tablespoon or two of carrier oil.

When you are dealing with recipes that are blended with a large volume of water or carrier oil there is no need to dilute further. For example, if you have four drops of lavender oil, two drops of geranium oil mixed with eight liters of water this will be fine for all sizes of pets.

Chapter 4 – Tips for successful application

Zoopharmacognosy of Essential Oils

Zoopharmacognosy is the branch of pharmacognosy that deals with animal self-medication. According to the principles of Zoopharmacognosy, the most effective technique of safe treatment of pets is allowing them to select essential oils they need and to direct you through the application process. Zoopharmacognosy argues that all pets have inborn ability to know the substances they need to consume to remain healthy. Hence, in the natural environment, a pet will select the minerals and herbs that will support its immune system, heal damaged cells and neutralize toxins.

Most probably, you have seen your pets eat grass from time to time. And if you observe them carefully, you will notice that they choose specific grasses. And even when the pet eats feces and dirt, it is looking for certain ingredients that can keep its body healthy. This is an act of self-medication. Therefore, even though you control the life of your pet, you should allow it to participate in selecting the right essential oils.

So what should you do to actualize Zoopharmacognosy in the care program for your pet? Give your pet the opportunity to pick the right essential oils by presenting the pet with a variety of oils. The good news is that if you make a huge variety of oils available to your pet, then you can simply stand aside and watch as it interacts with them and chooses the right one.

Indeed, as a rule, allow your pet to engage in choosing essential oils.

Use Essential Oils with Respect

Even though essential oils are natural, you should use them with knowledge, respect and the permission of your pet.

Before you even buy the oils, you should take your time to learn how they work Consult pet naturopathic experts and vets to advice you on the right choices. And just before applying the oil, make sure to dilute it thoroughly. Essential oils work best when diluted well.

But in all these, it is the respect you accord your pet that will boost the success of the therapy. Just like human beings need to be engaged respectfully by physicians, your pet deserves to be treated with dignity, and to participate in the selection of the essential oils. As a pet owner, therefore, you need to be patient with the pet and resist the temptation to rush things up because you think you know a lot better than the pet.

So how should you ensure that your pet feels respected? The secret is creating a connection with the pet so that an environment of security and safety emerges. The pet will always be relaxed as long as it feels the environment is safe.

Whenever your pet is anxious, especially when the anxiety or fear arises from the sight or smell of the oil you want to apply, make sure to calm the pet and to avoid rushing the application. To ensure that your pet is relaxed and feels safe:

Locate a spot in your home where the pet likes to rest. That must be the place the pet has identified as safer and more secure.

Lead the pet to that spot and sit quietly with it for some time, ignoring the pet for a while.

As you relax, gently begin to run your hands over your pet's fur, moving your hands from the back to the belly and then to the inside ears of the pet.

Continue to interact with the pet and allow connection to grow. Observe your pet's behavior and see whether it looks safe and secure.

With this connection, the pet will not find it strange to drink or smell essential oils when you bring oils to it.

Understand Your Pet's Responses

Understanding the responses of your pet to essential oils will really help you to achieve successful application. Every pet will show one of these four principal responses when confronted with essential oils:

Oral engagement: The pet will try to lick your hand or bottle of essential oil. To exploit this response for successful application, just add 3-4 drops of diluted oil in your hand and allow the pet to lick it.

Olfactory engagement: The pet will inhale deeply and then get into a trance with eyes flickering and nose twitching, or the pet will relax deeply in the area where the open bottle is located (and may just move away to a short comfortable distance). To exploit this response for successful application of essential oils, hold the open bottle so that the pet can smell the oil.

Indicative engagement: The pet will indicate to you the body area where it wants the oil to be rubbed, typically an acupressure point. Massage the point with the oil until the pet moves away.

Moving out of the range of the oil: When pets find oils unpleasant, they move far away. If this happens, respect the wishes of your pet and do not apply the oil further. Just imagine how you feel when you are smothered with a detestable fragrance and you have no good way of cleaning yourself except licking it off. And by remembering that your pet's sense of smell is 100x better than yours, you should respect its wishes when it finds the oil unpleasant.

Testing Your Pet's Responses

To know how your pet will respond to various essential oils, you should test the pet with the oils themselves. To do this successfully, you should:

Assess your pet's health condition so you can consider the most appropriate oils to use.

Make a list of oils that are effective in treating the condition of your pet.

Procure all the varieties of the oils and put them in closed bottles on the floor or just add drops of the oils to your hand, one at a time, and let your pet smell or lick the oils.

Observe how the pet responds to the oils.

For oils that are to be massaged on the skin dilute them well and then apply to the body, massaging and observing how the pet responds.

By testing your pet's responses to various oils, you can pick a list of oils that are both effective and acceptable to your pet, boosting the effectiveness of your treatment interventions.

Basic Precautions When Using Essential Oils with Pets

When using essential oils in pets, there are definitely a number of oils that must be avoided. Nevertheless, it is prudent to always consider the current condition of the pet and the degree of risk worth taking to save the pet's life. For example, if your pet has a severe kennel cough, you can use oregano or thyme because the risk taken is worth it. In fact, it is simply a matter of common sense when deciding when and what risks are worth taking. The basic safety rules for using essential oils with pets are:

Dilute oils ALWAYS with carrier oils such as olive oil or coconut oil. This reduces the risks immensely.

Avoid applying the oils on the nose, eyes, genital and anal areas. When using essential oils in pets, there are definitely a number of oils that must be avoided. Nevertheless, it is prudent to always consider the current condition of the pet and the degree of risk worth taking to save the pet's life. For example, if your pet has a severe kennel cough, you can use oregano or thyme because the risk taken is worth it. In fact, it is simply a matter of common sense when deciding when and what risks are worth taking. Besides, pets are MUCH SMALLER than humans; so you should make sure to apply MUCH LESS and MORE DILUTE oil than you would use with humans.

The basic safety rules for using essential oils with pets are:

- Dilute oils ALWAYS with carrier oils such as olive oil or coconut oil. This reduces the risks immensely.

- Avoid applying the oils on the nose, eyes, genital and anal areas.

- Take extreme caution when you use essential oils with very old, pregnant, or under 10-weeks old pets.

- Avoid using the following oils regularly: clove, thyme, wintergreen, camphor, oregano and cassia. These oils are not good for daily usage and should be used occasionally for severe illnesses such as kennel cough.

- Phototoxic essential oils should be used with care because they increase the risk of sunburn. Essential oils with high risks of sunburn include mandarin, bergamot, cumin, angelica, lovage, lime, grapefruit and lemon. Oils with lower risk of sunburn include Melissa, lemon verbena, ginger, cassia and caraway. When using these phototoxic oils make sure the pet is not exposed to sunlight soon after application.

- Prioritize therapeutic-grade and correctly-processed oils. Organic oils should be preferred over inorganic ones because they do not contain pesticides and other chemicals.

- When buying processed essential oils, go for cold-pressed ones because they allow natural properties and active ingredients to be properly expressed.

While the senses of our pets resemble our senses closely, their sense of smell greatly surpasses ours. For instance, an average pet has more than 200 million scent receptors while working pets have 230-300 million scent receptors. Humans only have 5 million scent receptors. Therefore, when administering essential oils to pets, you should consider this extremely powerful sense of smell and exploit it to achieve positive results.

Other tips for safe use of essential oils include:

Avoid using low-quality perfume-grade oils: Such oils are not safe for pets because most of them have not been properly grown, contain pesticides and are often adulterated with chemicals that may be toxic to pets.

Some essential oils are volatile and will ignite when exposed to flames or high temperatures. Therefore, do not leave diffusers or vaporizers unattended.

Never administer essential oils internally before you consult a vet or a pet naturopathic expert.

Be careful which oil you want to use directly on your pets skin. As a rule, dilute oils properly before application.

Avoid oils that can aggravate chronic conditions in pets already having those conditions.

Chapter 5 – Shopping guide for Essential oil

Apart from these essential items, you should also know the kind of effects the oil you are buying may have on your pet.

Find out whether the oil is applied topically, externally, aromatically or internally, and what level of dilution is necessary to avoid adverse effects. Also find out how the pet will be affected if exposed to the sun after the oil's application. Check the ingredient label carefully to see if the oil is designated as therapeutic grade. The label should indicate 100% essential oil, and it should clearly indicate the botanical name of the plant from which the oil has been extracted. For instance, if it is Clove Oil, the label will indicate Syzygium aromaticum. Remember to avoid oils whose labels indicate "Made from Natural Ingredients" or "Made with Essential Oils".

Essential oils can expire or become rancid. Therefore, when buying from a store, you should take note of the smell of the oil. Similarly, you should take note of the prices of various essential oil brands. Pure oils are never cheap and the more difficult the oil is to extract the costlier it is. Therefore, you should buy a reputable brand from a trustworthy dealer, without compromising on quality to get a cheaper brand.

Conclusion

There is still a lot that can be written when it comes to essential oils and pets but this book has all the basics that you need. As you start your journey into treating your pets naturally using essential oils, you will be amazed at how well they work.

You will soon be adept at reading your pet's visual cues when it comes to scents that they like and those that they really do not like. There is no need for concern here - most of the time, they will learn to enjoy their special aromatherapy time with you.

Best of all, your best friend will be able to enjoy a longer, happier life without resorting to noxious chemicals and products that really are not good for them.

Essential oils are easy and economical to use, highly effective and completely natural. It is simply a matter of choosing the right oils in the right concentrations, to use for the condition you are treating.

Once you have established what oils both you and your pet enjoy, look forward to a healthier pet!.

Finally, if you find this book helpful in any way, then I'd like to ask you for a friendly favor: Would you be nice enough to **leave an honest review** for this book on Amazon? I would love to know what you think. It'd be greatly appreciated. Thank you so much in advance!